CLEAN EATING: ESSENTIAL ONLY

Discover the Secrets to Health, Beautiful Body,
Youth and Longevity!

*«You will be amazed at how simple
it is to achieve with plenty of
new hacks and new facts...»*

BY
DEMI REESE

Table of Contents

Introduction

There is an increased likelihood that anyone who is concerned about their diet, health and fitness must have heard of "clean eating," as a concept and the numerous benefits that accompany it. But those who haven't heard about it might want to know what clean eating is all about? Where did it originate from? And what are its primary goals and objectives? Will it work for you?

It is essential for you to bear in mind as you read this book that it won't suggest any diet for you to follow, but will merely lay out the principles of clean eating in a very clear and concise manner so that you can adapt your dietary needs to it. This book does not give a detailed menu of Clean food because meal choices differ for each person. For instance, someone may like oatmeal for breakfast, while another could prefer scrambles or whole-grain pancakes. As a matter of fact, both choices are healthy and beneficial.

But the foremost thing is for you to understand the principles behind the formation of a healthy diet, that means what and when you need to eat. In addition to that, it should be seen as a flexible lifestyle that doesn't place any restriction on your dietary choices; for example, if you are a vegetarian, it means you can still enjoy your regular meals while holding on to the principles promoted by eating clean.

This book provides you with answers to all these questions because not only is it filled with priceless information and tips that will astonish you, but its content is entirely different from most boring books that you will find out there on healthy eating. It is designed to keep you engaged from the beginning to the end with compelling narratives that will leave a profound effect on you and will make your imaginations to run wild about clean eating.

Here, you will learn how to reprogram your conscious mind and have a smooth and efficient transition to clean eating. The overall idea behind this concept is to improve your quality of life in relation to your health, mood, appearance, and well-being in general. Also, people suffering from auto-immune diseases such as Celiac disease and inflammatory Bowel diseases like Chron's disease can significantly enjoy the benefits of following clean eating practices in order to manage their ailments.

At this juncture, it is crucial to emphasize that clean eating gives you the freedom and golden resources to find the right path to what really suits you as a person. Also, you must know that proper nutrition is not just about a diet, it is a way of life that should bring pleasure and satisfaction to you and your family!

Chapter One

The Emergence And Concept Of Clean Eating

Clean eating can be regarded as having the conviction that the consumption of whole foods that are as natural as possible and that staying away from foods that have been processed like refined sugar possesses immense health benefits for the body. To put it simply, it is about you having the conviction to stop feeding your body with junk!

Since it is a practical way of improving your overall standard of living, it is not surprising to find fitness gurus, nutritionists, and health-aware individuals to have been practicing this healthy eating technique for a very long time. It is pertinent to note at this stage that the term "clean eating" itself shouldn't be seen as a diet but as a way of life, which has always been in practice for millennia and even precedes the phrase itself.

Today, it is not uncommon to find Hollywood stars like Kate Perry lending credence to it and being devotees and promoters of this unique lifestyle. The idea of clean eating has always been linked to Ella Mills, Natasha Corrett, and the Hemsley sisters, even though they've all denied ever using the phrase. Several variants of it exist and might demand that you give up dairy products, gluten, grains and even promoting the consumption of food in its raw form.

The Principles Of Clean Eating

At first, it might appear as if it is a very difficult way of life for anybody to stick to, but on a closer look, you will discover that it is simple and straightforward to adopt its central beliefs. Some of the principles involved in clean eating include the following:

- Breakfast should be eaten within one hour of waking up in the morning every day
- To regulate blood sugar and put a stop to hunger, you ought to eat small regular meals about 5 times every day.
- Make sure that the foods you eat are whole foods; and that means they are not tampered with in their handling, packaging, and storage and are direct from the farm. For instance, fruits, legumes, vegetables, and grains must be whole; nuts and seed mustn't be salted, while chickens and beef must be reared free-range and grass-fed respectively.
- Your daily water intake should be at least 2 liters every day.
- Make sure there is an inclusion of healthy servings of lean protein, healthy fats and complex carbs in your meals.
- Steer clear of processed or refined foods like candies, sugar, white flour, white rice, etc
- Stay away from foods that are low in nutrition and packed full of calories, which in essence implies junk foods in every form.
- Drinks, sodas, and juices loaded with calories that do not have any nutritional value to your body should be avoided at all cost. Consider a scenario where someone is hooked to the harmful habit of taking at least a bottle of soda on a

daily basis and for many years. Now, reflect deeply on the damage substances like preservatives, and refined sugars may be causing to his/her health.

- Take advantage fresh fruits and vegetables to get fiber, vitamins, nutrients, and enzymes for your body.
- Manage the portions of every meal appropriately
- Avoid smoking and taking alcohol in excess quantity
- Try as much as possible to cook your meals.
- Perform routine exercise that will help you to stay fit and healthy
- Do not make food an object of worship
- Everything should be done in moderation.
- Don't become obsessed with it but try to live in pleasure.

Major Advantages Of Clean Eating

The crucial questions any health-conscious person may want to ask is what they stand to gain from clean food. Regardless of what your intentions or reasons are for wanting to adopt clean eating, you are going to find it to be a crucial and integral aspect of a wholesome lifestyle that will help boost your standard of living. Motives for wanting to eat clean could be driven by a desire to lose weight and live a healthy lifestyle or stay fit as you grow older.

Once you stick to wholesome and minimally unprocessed foods like fruits, nuts, seeds, fish, lean meat among several others, you will be providing your body with adequate nutrients to maintain healthy cell functions and to help combat chronic disease. Besides, when you take out unhealthful foods away from your meals, it provides enormous benefits as compounds discovered in harmful, and processed foods may raise your vulnerability to diseases.

The significant advantages of eating clean foods include the following:

- **To Boot Your Energy Levels**

Taking nutritious diets not only boost your energy levels and productivity but assist in nurturing your body correctly. A few nutrients that fuel your cells and enable them to work as they should, include B-complex vitamins and iron. Other benefits of eating clean are that it aids in the regulation of your blood sugar which, in turn, assist in putting a stop to spikes in blood sugar that could bring about exhaustion. And eating processed carbs like sweets often results in that type of health condition.

Quick Tip 1

An excellent way to get your energy levels going is to have breakfasts that consist of whole grains that are loaded with fibers, which will give you sufficient energy to take you through lunch.

Quick Tip 2

Foods that have been denatured or processed are often lacking in fiber, which aids in keeping stomach problems such as bloating and constipation under control. So eat healthy, fiber-rich foods to help keep constipation in check!

- **It Mitigate The Risks Of Cardiovascular Diseases**

When you opt for a lifestyle of taking clean, wholesome diet, you are, in some ways reducing the chances of suffering from cardiovascular disease. For example, vitamin C, a critical mineral that is present in fruits and vegetables in copious amount is known to strengthen the blood vessels; as a result, the intake of fruits and vegetables help lessen the possibility of having coronary heart disease and guard against high blood pressure or stroke.

It is essential to take into account the fact that certain healthy fat obtainable from plants such as olive, coconut and nuts tends to reduce unsafe cholesterol levels, which combats cardiovascular disease as well. Conversely, an unwholesome diet loaded with saturated fat raises your blood cholesterol, which puts your cardiovascular health at risk.

- **Combats Cancer**

Sticking to a clean diet offers tremendous assistance in the fight against the growth of cancer. It shouldn't come as a surprise to you that many studies have shown that a diet full of processed foods such as saturated fat, plant treated meat, and fried foods will increase your risk of having cancer.

Then again, a clean diet having sufficient amount of fruits and vegetables, enhances the ingestion of phytonutrients and antioxidants that crucial in fighting the growth of cancer.

Quick Tip 3

Adding plenty amount of cruciferous vegetables which are a family that comprises of broccoli, kale, tomatoes, etc. to your diet can be of assistance in the fight against the growth of cancer.

- **Plays A Vital Role In Maintaining Mental Health**

Aside from the vast benefits eating a clean diet provides to your physical well-being, it has been found to offer excellent support to your mental health as well. Certain nutrients found in a clean diet such as vitamin B-6 that are common in foods like banana and lean poultry aids in the production of dopamine, which plays a crucial role in the body feeling good and the elevation of your mood. In addition, essential nutrients like Omega-3 fatty acids have been found to sustain good mental health as well, so that a shortage of it in the body could result in glumness and depression.

Quick Tip 4

- Restricting your intake of caffeine may as well perk up your mental health because it can raise anxiety when taken in a significant amount.
- Furthermore, you need to avoid skipping meals as it may bring about stress, headache or tummy ache.

- **A Healthy Skin**

Eating clean to maintain a radiant skin and be healthy-looking is an age long practice that was even recorded in the Bible when the Jews were in exile in Babylon. Daniel and his friends had opted for a clean eating diet that consisted of fruits, beans, vegetables, and water as opposed to eating from the King's table. After the trial was over, Daniel and his friends were found to be healthier and more elegant in looks than their peers who had chosen to partake in meals from the King's table!

We can still draw on that vital lesson today because a lifestyle and diet that is free of processed foods, empty calories, refined sugar, and overindulgence in alcohol will certainly leave you with a radiant, glowing skin. The reason for it is because these unhealthful factors tend to deny the skin many useful nutrients it requires to stay strong and supple. Of course, you can nurture your skin to look fresher, healthy and young-looking with essential nutrients from the consumption of whole foods filled with skin-friendly nutrients like healthy fats and antioxidants.

- **You Get Unbelievable Flavor From Your Food**

Eating clean means, you will have meals that are reliant on a balanced mixture of foods that includes healthy proteins, carbohydrates, spices, and fats via natural foods. As soon as you start to cultivate this lifestyle, you will be amazed at how foods that are unprocessed taste, because you will be getting the actual flavor of natural foods.

Most foods in the traditional American diet are filled with chemicals like stabilizers, preservatives, sweeteners among several others, which tend to conceal the natural flavors of these foods. The resultant effect of these substances is that they are inclined to leave an aftertaste which may become noticeable when your taste buds become used to eating chemical-free, natural foods.

Aside from the increased energy levels, reduction in bloats, and the feel-good sensation you get from this lifestyle, you will discover that your food tastes better and nicer than you can ever imagine! It is worthy to note that as you indulge less in consuming junk foods, your desire to yearn for more of it will diminish significantly, and you will then discover the taste of real foods and be grateful for it.

- **Eating Clean Comes Cheap**

When compared to the huge dents that eating out at restaurants, having takeouts and chomping on junks leaves on your budget and wallets then you'll understand that making healthy appetizing meals at home not only comes cheap but is a far better option. In addition, with some excellent planning, you can get essential food items at your local farmers' market, natural foods store or co-op at a cheap rate thereby making your clean eating to come on the cheap.

- **Helps You To Cut Down Excess Weight**

When you combine the right work out routines, supplements, and along with all the huge benefits that are associated with clean eating, you will surely get that figure and shape you so much desire in little or no time.

Reasons Why It Will Work For You

Based on what has been established so far, there is no doubt that clean eating as a lifestyle is imbued with excellent health benefits, but what a lot of folks out there might want to know is if it is the "real deal," and would it work for them? Yes, it will work if you are determined to stick to the principles stated above because as stated earlier, clean eating centers its attention on taking balanced meals, managing the portion size of your meals, and doesn't outlaw any food groups. The following are additional reasons are why it should work for you:

- It doesn't seek to starve or deprive you of food but about adding healthy choices to your meals
- You will learn about making the correct food preferences
- The changes you need can be put into practice on any budget
- It seeks to empower and not make you feel gloomy
- Clean eating energizes you and makes you feel better
- Clean eating will make bloat to leave
- It will make you lose fat and shed excess weight
- Clean eating is a safe option for your family
- Since it is reliant on natural foods, then you will not be dealing with processed foods
- Clean eating is simply dependent upon common sense
- Clean eating is simple to implement
- Clean eating will make you discover the real taste of natural food!
- You will feel less hungry
- You are liable for the progress you make, and it holds you to account
- It is a lifestyle that will make you feel good!

Chapter Two

Transitioning To Clean Eating: A Step By Step Guide

Imagine a scenario where someone had been experiencing severe abdominal pains, gas, nausea, weight loss, nausea, and fatigue among several other indications and had just been diagnosed with Celiac disease. It is a chronic autoimmune disease, and s(he) had been advised by the physician to take to "clean eating," which requires observing a strict regimen of gluten-free diet. Yes, "clean eating," you heard right!

If the person described above is not conversant with such healthy eating lifestyle, s(he) may panic, go into a meltdown, and start thinking that the world is about to come to an end. The cheering news for them is that evolution to Clean Eating must be devoid of stress, and the entire course of action is supposed to give them a great deal of excitement and pleasure.

Although there is bound to be challenges along the way, such as your body resisting the changes taking place with your eating practices and some pains that may go with it. You should see it as an avenue for you to learn new things, view life from a different perspective and as a participant from the other side too. It is essential for anybody wishing to take to clean eating to follow the steps given below:

- **Identify "Why" You Want To Go On This Journey**

Taking up the new habit of clean eating requires a great deal of effort; therefore you must reflect deeply on what is motivating and driving you to want to embark on this journey. It could be that you are suffering from a medical condition that could be remedied by sticking to a clean diet or maybe you are planning to get yourself in good shape for an impending sporting event. Perhaps you are beginning to feel concerned that all your past unhealthful misdemeanors are about catching up on you and you are really troubled about the lasting health effects they may have such that you feel like making atonement for it and to live a healthy life from thereon.

All the scenarios cited above are sufficient reasons for anybody to desire a cleaner change in diet. The most excellent incentive to instigate transformation must come from within the individual and is entrenched in positive thinking.

- **Find Out How Much Time You Are Prepared To Give**

Forming new habits with life-changing goals can take some time that could slide into some months or more. Having established your **"why,"** it is imperative you decide how much time you are ready to give to the process of planning your food, shopping for groceries, and cooking your meals. Whichever way you look at it, moving towards a really clean diet is bound to be a long-term goal for nearly everybody.

Quick Tip 5

You could choose to give up your favorite Saturday night TV show to prepare healthy breakfasts that would last for a full week.

- **Carry Out A Detailed Assessment Of Your Present Diet**

By employing the use of a food journal, you can keep track of what you have been eating so far, and to enable you to review what needs to be added and what you can reduce from your existing diet. Having gotten data for your analysis, you will have to make out emerging patterns from your samples and then draw up two lists that would contain:

- Foods which aren't so healthy that you will like to cut down from your diet; however, if you have a lengthy list of such foods then you may select around 3-5 apparent references such as sugar-laden foods, sodas and unhealthy snacks that you'd love to take care of initially.

- Secondly, you'd have to itemize a list of wholesome foods which are absent in your existing schedule. Remember that the goal of clean eating is to lay emphasis on taking nutrient-rich foods and not just reducing the junks. Also, you will have to take into account the number of vegetables on your list, and if there are any shortcomings, then you can add a few veggies to it for the next shopping.

- **Be Practical In Selecting Your Targets**

After you've decided on the unnutritious foods that you want to do away with on your schedule and the beneficial ones you'd like to include in your diet; afterward you will have to put together a few strategic choices. An excellent and useful way to go about this is to set several small goals that you can always work on; it is a lot better than making an effort to engage the whole thing right away. That way, they can tally up fast. The crucial questions you'd need to take into account include; what modifications are likely going to give you the highest probability of success? Which of the small clean eating practices do you intend to go for initially? At the beginning of a new month, simply add from there.

- **Set SMART Objectives And Write Them Down**

It is essential you set objectives that are **SMART** (specific, measurable, achievable, realistic and has a timescale). For instance, let's say you want to tackle your obsession with unhealthy double fried donuts. Maybe you eat about 4 pieces every day, and then it becomes necessary you set vital parameters about your objectives as given below.

First, you may need to define your goal by making a statement that is reliant on self-control and then stating that: "I am going to stop taking many donuts."

The statement above is not specific in its objective and lacks other vital parameters as well; for instance, it doesn't spell out the number of donuts allowed each day, if there is going to be any at all so that you'll have to revise the statement further to the following:

"I am going to cut down my donut intake to **2** each day for the next **one week.** Afterward, I will reduce it to one donut the **following week** and stop taking donuts completely in the **third week.** Should I have the urge to eat donuts, I will resort to healthy homemade snacks (preferably fruits and vegetables) that have been stocked up in my refrigerator and drink plenty of water along with it to satisfy my cravings."

Now, the above statement has given **measurable** and **specific** objectives by stating the number of donuts you are going to cut down each week, the **timeline** for you to achieve your objectives and even provide healthy substitutes or alternatives to make your goals **realistic** and **achievable.** All you need to do is to put in the hard work to make it possible.

As a result, there is no vagueness in the above proclamation. It simply gives you a clear path that will allow you to control your cravings.

The last step is for you to write down your goals and if possible stick them on the walls of your bedroom or kitchen as a reminder of the task before you.

- **Read The Nutrition Labels**

Learning to read what is on food labels is a critical aspect of clean eating since they allow you to find out virtually everything that you need to know regarding what you are about to put in your stomach. Remember that not all products in boxes or packages are detrimental to your health, so it is essential you examine all the ingredients on the labels to enable you to make the best decision. There are some simple rules about labels that you need to follow if you must eat clean and they include:

- Focus on foods with labels that consist of words like, "modified," "refined," "hydrolyzed."
- Also, you'll have to watch out for those that point to additional processing and words that end in "-ose," as they signify the addition of sugars, and a common pattern is the word "fructose."
- Try to find labels with words like "gluten-free," "whole grains" and "whole wheat" in the ingredients. However, don't buy them just because you have those phrases stamped on them, it is best you do your research about them and go to stores that are renowned for natural and minimally processed foods.

- Ensure that foods with high calories have the bulk of the calories coming from fiber and proteins.
- Make sure the level of sodium, saturated fat and sugar on the labels are as low as possible.
- The ingredients on the labels must be rather few and reflect on every one of them by asking yourself this honest question, "Do I really want this ingredient in my kitchen and inside my body." If your answer is not affirmative, then you'll have to drop it and move on. In fact, if the ingredients on your label number more than five, it advisable to drop it as there is no way you'd want them in your cart, kitchen, and tummy!
- If there is an ingredient on the label that you don't understand, the chances are that you are dealing with a highly processed food, and then you'll have to think about putting it back on the shelf.
- To gauge if foods are closer to nature, you should view them from the perspective of sea, land, and trees.
- If your label reads like a science experiment, then you ought not to eat something from it.

Personally, if I want to take some ice cream, I'll go for the ones that are low in carb, chemical free and contain just four ingredients which are cream, milk, egg yolks, and sugar.

Quick Tip 6

Reading labels to examine the ingredients list on them is essential because at times, 'organic' and 'natural' might be misleading.

- **Buy In Large Quantities**

Your clean eating program will only gain traction if you are able to get grocery stores with produce and freezer sections to buy food items in bulk. Getting such a store will allow you to fill your freezer with all the fruits, vegetables, beef, chickens, etc. you need, and also grant you immediate access to ready-made meals. It is possible to make purchases of items in bulk on the internet as well.

Quick Tip 7

Buying food items in bulk saves you two essential commodities which are time and money (fantastic discounts often go with them), and they are some of the reasons why eating clean is a far cheaper lifestyle!

You also have the option of buying some of your foods on the internet too.

- **Place Emphasis On A Meal Or Snack At A Time**

As stated earlier, it is crucial you take it one meal at a time, instead of focusing on making wholesale changes that could overwhelm you and your family in the long run. Start by taking a meal or snack and make them clean by adding clean substitutes like replacing corned beef with grass-fed beef. In no time, you'd have cleaned the meal entirely and taken out all the unhealthful choices.

Bear in mind that your family may not like the changes at first, but be firm and they will get used to the alterations you made gradually. Enlighten members of your family as to why you are trying to clean the meals and make them understand that it not just another diet, but as an enduring arrangement that's meant to make them strong and healthy. But don't do away with all their favorite foods at once!

- **Go Organic!**

Is it really worth the cost? That is a common question people often ask when advised to take to organic foods. However, when you evaluate the long-term health benefits of eating organic foods against the price, then you'll know that it is really worth every penny paid for them. What do you stand to gain from eating organic foods?

- Organic foods are toxin free which, in essence, means no pesticide, herbicides and any chemical during planting, harvesting, handling, and storage. Although it is not realistic to have all foods as organic but it is necessary for you to have some organic foods like Apples, Peaches, Grapes, Celery, Potatoes, Cherry tomatoes, etc.
- GMOs (genetically modified organisms) are prohibited in all stages of growing or producing and processing organic foods.
- As stated earlier, organic foods are chemical-free and save consumers the burden of having to ingest residues of chemicals on foods. For instance, tons of chemicals are used in America yearly on crops that are not grown organically. So when you eat organic, you are eating chemical-free foods.

- Two fats that are good for the heart, CLA (conjugated linoleic acid) and omega-3 fatty acids are usually found in high amount in organically reared meat and milk and can significantly enhance the health of your heart.
- Organic foods are good for pregnant, and nursing mothers as chemicals from foods not grown organically are known to get to the child during breastfeeding and at the stage of pregnancy.
- Without a doubt, organic foods are better for children as it aids in significantly lowering their exposure to the pesticide, and hence reducing the levels of chemicals in their body as well.
- There is no disputing the fact that organically grown foods taste better than those grown with chemicals.
- It makes the rearing of strong and productive organic livestock possible, because the animals have access to excellent nutrition and are raised without antibiotics, and growth hormones.

Quick Tip 8

Organic foods are usually stocked at the perimeter of the grocery store, and you are likely to find whole grains, fresh fruits, meats, seafood, etc. at this point.

Processed foods are often located right in the store itself!

- **Cook Your Meals**

Preparing your meals allows you gain control over what goes into your body and it isn't surprising that homemade meals taste better and are more hygienic than foods cooked at eateries. Cooking your meals offers you tremendous benefits that include:

- You can manage the amount of salt, sugar, flavors, and fats that you put in your meals.
- It saves you the agony of restaurant foods that often contain plenty of sodium, salt, and butter in almost everything they prepare.
- It is a chance to let your children partake in the cooking process because they can include a fruit or vegetable of their choice into every meal. You can't trade the pleasure they get from eating what they've added from the grocery store or kitchen for anything in this world!
- Cooking your meals allow you to experiment with a broad range of things like throwing in some vegetables when you feel like having some or sneaking some mushrooms in place of steaks!
- The simpler the food, the better. Eat simple and Eat clean should be your dictum at all times.

Quick Tip 9

To draw out the natural taste and sweetness of veggies like carrots, potatoes, onions, and parsnip among several others, you should consider roasting them!

Chapter Three

Having The Right Attitude To Clean Eating

Once you've made up your mind to practice clean eating, it is essential that you develop the right approach not only to yourself but the world around you as well. For instance, one critical aspect is how you will manage your cravings for junk food since old habits hardly die. This chapter deals with ways to approach clean eating as a lifestyle and some crucial guides to help you put the problems you might encounter in check as soon as you choose to take a bold step towards it.

Ways To Combat Cravings

It is not unusual for unhealthful habits like longing for sugar or carbohydrates from your previous lifestyle to come back to haunt you while attempting to stick to a clean eating system. It is advisable you don't avoid them totally; however, you mustn't go over the top with it. The 80% principle comes into play here, because as soon as you've gotten to your objective of making clean eating a lifestyle and you are able to maintain it about 80% of the time then it becomes tolerable to give yourself a treat once in a while. You can combat cravings by taking the following steps:

- First, start by gulping a glass of water and see if the longing leaves. But if doesn't then you may try the following tips below.
- For example, you could make a healthy plant fat like avocado pear handy, along with several proteins. Eating a small piece of fish or meat with the avocado pear would do

the trick of satisfying your yearnings and keep you going for an extended period.

- Also, you may flavor your vegetables and foods with unrefined sea salt, which lack calories and doesn't put your health at significant risk.
- An idle mind they say is the Devil's workshop! So put a stop to the allure of those unhealthy, but scrumptious images of junks running riots in your head by keeping your mind busy with a simple walk around your neighborhood or do some work in the garden.
- Go outside and enjoy spending time with nature as the warm rays of the sun and fresh breeze caress your skin.
- Without being fanatical about eating clean, you should avoid trying to impose harsh restrictions on yourself regarding something you crave. As stated earlier, you can afford to take some of your favorite snacks, but in small quantities, and not all in one day. Discipline should be your watchword!
- Again, if the urge to have your favorite chocolate becomes too much that you can't even resist it, and then you may decide to eat half portion of it along with something healthy. Otherwise, you can reject it outrightly.

Snacks

When buying or preparing your snacks, there are some things that you need to take into account, and they include the following:

- Although they don't have to be combined in an ideal proportion, the presence of healthy fats, proteins, and a few carbohydrates are indispensable. Moreover, you can take a snack with any combination of two out of the three; however, you'll have to steer clear of snacks containing only carbohydrates.

- Perhaps you are considering a snack of fruits; it won't be out of place if you take some fat and protein with it. The function of fat and protein is to make you feel full quickly, satisfied and then stop the longings.

- Fresh, green vegetables are entirely okay for you to snack on, all through the day.

- It is essential to remember that having nibbles isn't compulsory, so there is no point in going for one if you don't have the urge.

Tips For Mindful Eating

A busy way of life makes it crucial that you take bites of food in between tasks, but when you opt to eat clean, you'd have to put that habit aside and focus on your food. In that case, imbibing some practices of being mindful of what you eat is essential. Mindful eating simply means no consumption of food in front of the TV; while sitting behind your desk or computer; inside the vehicle, and while standing. To make you remain motivated and focused on your objectives, you can use some positive mantras to ward off negative thoughts.

Quick Tip 10

You can make use of small plates to control and manage the size of your meals. Take your meals on salad plates and utilize little bowls to eat cereals and soups. Play on your mind by tricking it into believing you have more food. After all, the same size of food will look smaller on a big plate with spaces around it!

Chapter Four

Clean Eating On A Budget: Things You Need To Know!

A lot of people are very much aware of the benefits of clean eating and would want to clean their meals, but they are often deterred by the widespread notion that it is a lifestyle that can be pricey to maintain. Indeed, eating clean meals might be a drain on your financial resources if you allow it.

However, this chapter seeks not only to dispel the myth that healthy nutrition is expensive and difficult but addresses pertinent issues relating to living a clean eating lifestyle without you having to break the bank. You will get incredible tips that are easy to execute and will help you save some hard earned cash, while you are still able to enjoy your clean eating system. More like eating your cake and having it back!

Do Your Research

Before heading to the grocery store, it is vital that you carry out your research on what you'll be looking out for when you go shopping. You must know the concept of reading labels correctly and be familiar with the need to avoid processed foods, chemical additives, and refined sugars.

Draw Up A Shopping List And Develop A Meal Plan

Plan, plan, plan and be strategic in your planning. The significance of a shopping list can't be exaggerated, but it even becomes vital to the success of any clean eating routine when you take into account the fact that it can assist in reducing cost, especially once you focus on fresh produce that is on sale in season.

Again, you may choose to take into consideration recipes with related ingredients that are used all through the week to avoid wasting your food items. For example, a meal consisting of potato such as sweet potato bowl may crop up on Tuesday and then you choose to add another potato dish by the weekend with choice proteins and fats to go with it!

Quick Tip 11

Planning your shopping simply helps in time management and reducing wastes!

Avoid Shopping On A Hungry Tummy

When you make this mistake and go shopping hungry, then there is a high tendency that the hankering for food will result in you making impulsive buys and even blur your decision-making ability. Some healthy nibblings choices like almond nuts with plenty of water won't do you any harm should you start feeling hunger pains before going shopping.

Focus On In-Season Produce And Watch Out For Sales

The prices of produce are likely to go down during the time of harvest, and it is the period when the tastes of foods hit the highest point in regards to flavor and nutrient. For instance, the summer months are the best time to get fruits like apricots, cherries, and melons among several others.

You can join many clean eating groups on the internet that are living close to your area to glean information about scheduled sales from them and then plan your meals based on what you are likely to get from there. Tweaking your meals to be flexible with the availability of produce during such seasons will certainly save you some good dough!

Check Other Shopping Venues For Excellent Deals

Even though you may have your favorite grocery store where you do your shopping, there is still need for you to explore other avenues for better deals. You'd be surprised at what your adventure will yield, after trying out other places like the local farmers' markets where you can gain access to some cheap, fresh, and clean produce.

Buy A Slow Cooker

To make the preparation of clean, healthy food easier and faster, you should consider buying a slow cooker.

Buy Foods In Bulk

This factor has been explained in chapter two and can be a terrific money-saver in the sense that it saves you time when you make bulk purchases of commonly used items like fruits, vegetables, grains, spices, legumes while enjoying fantastic discounts along with it.

Know When To Go Organic

Some crops like onions, maize, avocado pear, sweet potatoes, mangoes, kiwi, cabbages, etc. tend to soak up a negligible amount of chemicals during production and are usually acceptable if you go for them when grown conventionally. As a result, you don't have to worry if the money to buy them organically isn't sufficient!

Freeze Your Foods After Storing Them Correctly

Eating clean on a budget warrants that you cultivate the habit of saving your fruits, vegetables, and proteins correctly. Not doing that could bring about wastage which is not an outcome you'd wish for. Make sure you organize your refrigerator very well and take advantage of airtight, reusable containers for storing certain fruits and vegetables. Moreover, you could find some retailed produce at great discounts that you can then store up in your freezer.

Be Creative With Leftovers

Make use of leftovers creatively by integrating them into subsequent dishes you prepare or as go-to meals the following day.

Experiment With Ingredients In Your Fridge

As weird as this may sound, you would be amazed at how tasty, certain combinations of fruits, vegetables and spices could be if you just throw them into your preferred whole grain in a stir fry and along with a dash of salt.

Go Shopping With A Friend

It's best if you go shopping with a friend who shares your clean eating ideals because you are not only going to have fun shopping but will enjoy discounts, split some costs and fresh produce as well. Besides, it reduces the likelihood of you wasting food since you are not going to buy in excess of what you have need of.

Chapter Five

The Proteins, The Fats, And The Carbs!

Proteins, fats, and carbohydrates are macronutrients and can be regarded as the fundamental building blocks of clean eating. They form the basis of a balanced diet and are needed by the body in a significant amount for growth, metabolism, and other bodily functions. It is crucial you understand how they work because the body must get them in the right combination and amount to function properly. Having a balanced diet doesn't mean you have to focus on restricting specific foods, but it is all about adding the proper macronutrients to the body and in the right form too.

Proteins

Protein plays a crucial role in the growth and in equally building and sustaining lean muscle tissue that in turn, enhances the metabolism of the body. Its benefits to the body include the following:

- Protein has a role to play in regulating enzymes and hormones.
- It is concerned with the fixing of tissues and growth, and to maintain lean muscle tissue too.
- Protein is vital in building essential hormones and enzymes in addition to immune function.
- Protein assists the body in secreting the hormone glucagon that acts to oversee insulin and keep its levels under control.
- Protein serves as a secondary energy source when carbs/glucose is not accessible.
- Protein maintains the growth and health of the skin, hair, and nails.

Quick Tip 12

You should up your intake of proteins if you want a lean look with abs!

Fat

Fat is a key source of fuel and offers two times the energy of carbohydrates or protein in the body. The reason is that dietary fat has more calories per gram and has more than twice the calories you are likely to get from carbs or protein of the same weight. Fats shouldn't be seen as an enemy because taking healthy fats will assist you in controlling your attempt to lose weight by giving you a better feeling of satiety than when you consume foods low in fat. As a result, it is easier for you to avoid overeating because your body sensibly informs you that you are full already. Other benefits of fats include:

- It is crucial for growth and development plus sustaining cell membranes and serving as a cushion for internal organs.
- Fats assist the body in absorbing certain vitamins and carotenoids.
- It helps to lubricate the joints.
- It aids in maintaining a healthy skin and hair.
- It enlivens and makes food taste better.
- Fat assist in holding back longings for food because it gives a sense of satisfaction.

Some healthy fats for your clean eating include Coconut oil, olive oil, and butter, in particular, clarified butter.

Carbohydrates

Carbs are a foremost source of energy to the body. Carbohydrates fuel our activities and are the chief energy source for muscle function. In the body, carbs are broken-down to enable it to get glucose, which is utilized for energy and to also give the body essential fiber, vitamins, and minerals as well. Attributes of carbs are not limited to the following:

- "Bad carbs" are mostly processed foods like sugar, white bread, sugary cereals and are digested easily and swiftly in the body. Their digestibility results in spikes in the blood glucose levels, which in turn, causes insulin levels in the body to experience a similar movement thereby leading to tiredness in the individual. They can significantly harm your weight loss effort because they can impact adversely on your metabolism.

- On the other hand, complex carbohydrates are regarded as "good carbs" because they are rich in fiber and are slow to digest by the body when eaten. They serve as a slow-burning reservoir of energy that keeps the body going and also makes the body full for a more extended period. This type of carbohydrate will improve your weight loss effort. Examples include whole grains, beans, seeds legumes, several fruits, and starchy vegetables among several others.

Quick Tip 13

In the absence of a scale when planning your meals, you can carry out measurements with your bare hands in the following ways:

- Use your palm or fist to measure proteins
- Again, use palm or fist to measure cooked starchy carbohydrates
- Measure fats with the size of your thumb
- The quantities of Veggies are limitless!

Chapter Six

Clean Eating For Fitness And Longevity

There is no disputing the fact that taking the right type of food plays a significant role in helping people sustain a longer and healthier life. Still, several factors tend to restrict many individuals from making the right food choices that will be of benefit to them, especially as they grow older.

Some of the reasons could be partly due to a lack of appetite, difficulties cooking meals, not liking a particular fruit or vegetable and sometimes due to ignorance. Research has shown that finding the right food that you desire, and eating them in the right amount is the secret to living a healthy and long life. Some few practical steps may be of help here:

- Older folks should consider splitting their calorie intake into proteins for your muscles, calcium for the development of bones, and an essential heart-friendly diet which can assist in putting excess weight in check. The reason is that many old people are obese and are prone to conditions like heart disease, diabetes, etc.
- The reduction of calories in the meals of animals to some degree has been proven to prolong their life while this concept can be adapted to humans, but it should be done in moderation.
- Although proteins, in general, are known to lower mortality rate, plant protein has been found to be of more benefit than animal protein. On the other hand, animal protein like

chicken and fish has been found to be better than red or processed meat in diet.

The following list of food should enhance your longevity:

Spice: There is a range of spices to bring your food to life, and they are an excellent source of antioxidants. Also, they are imbued with plenty of anti-inflammation, anticancer and anti-obesity attributes.

Proteins: Add proteins to your diet in the right amount and combination.

Dark leafy green veggies: There are some nutrient dense dark leafy green vegetables with lower calories and should be part of your diet. They also protect the brain from the adverse impact of aging.

Eat more fiber: Fibre rich-foods like oatmeal, whole wheat, and cereals help in the movement of the bowels and the regulation of blood sugar.

Nuts: Nuts like walnuts make healthy snacks and helps in regulating blood sugar spikes and is a great boost to living longer.

Adopt a Mediterranean diet: Research has shown that people who stick to this diet live longest on earth. You'd have to eat chicken, fish; fruits, olive oil and plenty of fruits and veggies to enable you to harness the benefits of this diet.

Incorporate good bacteria into your diet: Fermented foods such as yogurt, kefir, natto, sauerkraut, and kimchi have probiotics that help prolong our lifespan. Have you ever wondered why Japan has some of the oldest people in the world? It just has a lot to do with the fermentation of their foods.

Movement Is Life

The secret of longevity is to be active by moving all through the day. You should engage in physical exercise and sports that will help you maintain your fitness. An exercise that you can find useful is the NEAT (Non-exercise activity thermogenesis) because it focuses on activities you can perform and integrate into your daily routine that will be beneficial in the long term. It is known to be of more value than the regular exercise habits you are used to doing because it helps you to:

- Cut down excess fat
- Energize you
- Prevent diabetes and several other chronic diseases
- Enhance your energy levels
- Speed up our metabolism
- Ultimately prolonge your lives

Conclusion

We have highlighted the origin, benefits and transiting to clean eating while providing amazing tips on ways you can eat clean on a budget. Furthermore, we took a look at the building blocks of a healthy meal which are proteins, carbohydrates, and fats. Lastly, we talked about clean eating towards a healthy lifestyle and longevity, while emphasizing the need to moderate calorie intake and the consumption of animal protein. The importance of physical activities that include all kinds of routines and sport cannot be overstated.

Don't be afraid to be a little better. Just take the first step into a new **active life**. Once you try it, you'll never be the same again. First of all, you'll change the attitude to yourself. Believe me, it's addictive ... Let yourself live more interesting, healthier, longer ...

Isn't this what everyone wants?